ILEOSTOMY DIET COOKBOOK

I0429946

Delicious And Nutrient-Packed Friendly Recipes For Body Nourishment, Easy Digestion And Elevating Your Health

DR LUCAS KAYCE

DISCLAIMER

This book about illness and nutrition is not meant to replace expert medical advice, diagnosis, or treatment; rather, it is meant purely for informational reasons. This book's content is founded on broad concepts and recommendations for managing diseases and nutrition.

Before adopting any major dietary or lifestyle changes, readers are recommended to speak with a qualified healthcare provider, such as a licensed physician or registered dietitian, especially if they have pre-existing medical concerns. Everybody has different health demands, so what works for one person might not work for another.

The use of the information provided in this book may have unfavorable repercussions or consequences, for which the author and publisher disclaim all liability. No disease is meant to be identified, treated, cured, or prevented by the information provided.

The book may include contain references to medical literature or research findings; however readers are urged to independently confirm this material and contact reliable sources.

It is important to remember that the fields of nutrition and medicine are always changing, and that new findings could have an impact on the advice offered in this book. As a result, readers are urged to keep up with the most recent advancements in healthcare and, when in doubt, seek professional counsel.

By reading this book, readers agree that they are in charge of their own health decisions and release the author and publisher from any liability arising from the use of the material in the book, whether direct or indirect.

TABLE OF CONTENTS

ABOUT THE BOOK

For those managing their lives with an ileostomy, the "Ileostomy Diet Cookbook" is an invaluable resource. This book, a crucial resource in the field of health and wellness discusses the particular dietary difficulties that come with having an ileostomy and offers helpful advice as well as a plethora of information for keeping a healthy, balanced diet.

The cookbook is methodically organized, providing readers with a thorough grasp of ileostomy fundamentals, tips for designing an ileostomy-friendly kitchen, and dietary recommendations catered to the unique requirements of ileostomy patients.

Starting with an overview of what an ileostomy is, the book explores the practical aspects of everyday life and the nutritional concerns that are important for those adjusting to this life-changing experience. After that, readers are taken step-by-step through the process of establishing an ileostomy-friendly kitchen, with a focus on how important it is to use basic cooking utensils and stock the pantry with the correct products. The nutritional suggestions that follow address subjects including vitamin and mineral requirements, hydration advice, and nutrient balancing. They are carefully designed to provide readers with the knowledge they need to maintain a well-balanced diet.

The "Ileostomy Diet Cookbook" is mostly composed of tasty and varied recipes that are thoughtfully arranged into categories for each meal of the day. From healthy one-pot dinners to vibrant breakfast dishes, the cookbook offers a variety of options to suit a range of palates and dietary requirements. Snacks, sides, desserts, and special occasion recipes are all included to make sure that people with ileostomies can have a varied and fulfilling food experience.

Additionally, the book expands on its practical advice to cover social issues, including advice on how to plan special occasions, organize ileostomy-friendly gatherings, and deal with the difficulties of traveling and eating out.

With this all-encompassing approach, the "Ileostomy Diet Cookbook" becomes a holistic lifestyle guide for anyone looking to live a satisfying and health-conscious life with an ileostomy, rather than just a compilation of recipes.

WELCOME TO THE COOKBOOK FOR THE ILEOSTOMY DIET

Welcome to the Ileostomy Diet Cookbook, where we will take you on a trip to discover the complex relationship between ileostomy and nutrition, illuminating the dietary factors that are vital to ileostomy patients' overall health.

This cookbook functions as a thorough guide, providing not only a plethora of mouthwatering recipes but also insightful information about how ileostomy affects dietary requirements.

An ileostomy is a surgical technique in which the ileum, or lower portion of the small intestine, is diverted through a stoma, or abdominal orifice. Many medical disorders, including inflammatory bowel disease, colon cancer, and congenital anomalies, necessitate this life-altering surgery.

Changes in the digestive tract affect how waste is eliminated and how nutrients are absorbed by those who have an ileostomy.

COMPREHENDING DIETARY CONSIDERATIONS AND ILEOSTOMY

Comprehending the subtleties of an ileostomy is essential for customizing a diet that promotes general well-being and minimizes possible difficulties. Water, electrolyte, and vitamin absorption are all impacted by the digestive tract's rerouting through the stoma, which modifies the natural digestive process. For those who have an ileostomy, keeping a diet that is nutrient-dense and well-balanced is crucial to preventing deficits and fostering optimal health.

For those who have an ileostomy, diet is more than just selecting what to eat; it also entails planning for possible obstacles. Prioritizing foods that are readily digested and unlikely to irritate or produce blockages around the stoma is common.

The cookbook explores these issues and provides advice on how to choose foods and create recipes that are not only tasty but also easy on the stomach.

The Ileostomy Diet Cookbook highlights the significance of customizing meals to meet specific needs since dietary tolerance varies across individuals. It acknowledges the variety of dietary choices and attempts to offer a flexible selection of dishes to suit various palates and cultural contexts. The cookbook aims to stimulate culinary creativity by offering a variety of dishes, from creative appetizers to filling main meals, all of which are tailored to meet the specific dietary needs of those who have ileostomies.

This cookbook is a comprehensive resource that fosters awareness of ileostomy and provides useful strategies for overcoming food obstacles, rather than merely a list of meals.

CHAPTER ONE

BASICS OF ILEOSTOMY

DESCRIBE ILEOSTOMY

An ileostomy is a surgical operation in which an incision is made in the abdominal wall to bring the ileum—a section of the small intestine—to the surface. This type of surgery is usually carried out when a section of the colon or rectum has to be removed or bypassed because of congenital problems, colorectal cancer, or inflammatory bowel disease. With an ileostomy, waste can be removed from the body by a different pathway, with digestive juices leaving the body through the stoma—a surgically made abdominal orifice. Ileostomies come in a variety of forms, such as loop and end, and each fulfills a distinct set of medical requirements.

MAINTAINING AN ILEOSTOMY

Living with an ileostomy necessitates adapting to major physical and psychological changes in one's everyday routine. People who have an ileostomy frequently struggle with issues of self-esteem, body image, and the day-to-day care of their stoma.

For patients to successfully navigate the initial phase of adaptation, healthcare providers must provide them with the necessary education and assistance. A proper pouching system, appropriate ostomy supplies, and knowledge of how to care for the stoma are essential components of everyday ileostomy maintenance.

HANDLING NUTRITIONAL DIFFICULTIES

For those who have an ileostomy, managing nutritional problems is one of the most important factors. People may have alterations in their ability to digest food and absorb nutrients since an ileostomy bypasses a section of the digestive tract.

It becomes essential to keep up a diet that is readily digested and well-balanced to avoid potential problems including electrolyte imbalances, starvation, and dehydration.

Physicians frequently advise a gradual return of foods to the diet so that patients can learn which meals can cause problems with their ileostomy output.

The effects of an ileostomy on digestion can be controlled with certain dietary adjustments. Soluble fiber, drinking plenty of water, and chewing meals well all help promote easier digestion.

It is recommended that people who have an ileostomy stay away from specific foods that could cause more gas, stink, or blockages. Speaking with a certified dietitian or other medical expert can also offer tailored advice on food selections to maximize nutrition while having an ileostomy.

An ileostomy is a surgical surgery that results in a stoma to eliminate waste and adjust to life with one needs both mental and physical changes. Choosing the right supplies, changing one's lifestyle, and providing appropriate stoma care are all essential components of effective ileostomy care.

Handling dietary difficulties is an important factor that requires well-balanced, readily digestible food in addition to medical specialists' advice to guarantee the best nutrition and general health for people who have an ileostomy.

CHAPTER TWO

THE KITCHEN APPROPRIATE FOR ILEOSTOMY

PUTTING FOOD IN YOUR PANTRY

Any effective and efficient kitchen must include a well-stocked pantry, especially for people managing life with an ileostomy. The secret to success is to have a healthy mix of necessities that address nutritional requirements as well as the unique dietary needs related to ileostomies.

Make sure you have a range of low-residue and easily digested-foods available first. White rice, spaghetti, canned fruit, and thoroughly cooked veggies may be examples of this.

Choose products that are canned or jarred and have fewer additives and preservatives; these can be easier on the stomach. A well-rounded diet should include nutrient-rich foods such as broth and canned proteins (tuna, chicken).

For ileostomy patients, managing fiber is essential; limit consumption of whole grains or high-fiber cereals and opt for refined grains instead. Rice cakes, smooth nut butter, and low-fiber crackers are a few possible snack options. It's also a good idea to remember to stay hydrated; electrolyte-rich drinks or sports drinks can assist in restoring vital nutrients that are lost due to increased fluid output.

For those who have an ileostomy, maintaining a healthy digestive tract is very vital, so think about using shelf-stable probiotics to enhance gut health. Make sure everything in your cupboard is within its expiration date by regularly reviewing and updating it, and keep an eye out for any new dietary requirements.

CRUCIAL UTENSILS FOR THE KITCHEN

Having the appropriate kitchenware can help you streamline your cooking and adjust to the special difficulties that come with following an ileostomy-friendly diet. To prepare meals efficiently, start with a strong cutting board and sharp knives. Given the prevalence of canned products, a can opener is essential, and a silicone spatula makes it easier to remove the last bit of food from cans or jars.

Invest in non-stick cookware to reduce the amount of additional fat that is needed when cooking. For smooth purees or adding easily digested items to meals, a food processor or blender can be quite helpful. Measuring tools are essential for accurate portion management and rigorous adherence to dietary requirements for people with certain dietary restrictions.

To avoid cross-contamination, set aside specific kitchenware and tools just for ileostomy-friendly meal preparation. It's crucial to keep a clean and well-maintained kitchen for people with weakened digestive systems.

Adaptable storage containers keep ingredients accessible and tidy, whether they are perishable or non-perishable. Finally, it's a proactive move to keep an emergency kit stocked with materials for handling unforeseen ileostomy-related circumstances.

TIPS FOR MEAL PLANNING

The foundation of running an ileostomy-friendly kitchen is meal planning, which gives nutritional decisions structure and consistency. Start by creating a weekly food plan that includes a variety of nutrients and takes into consideration any dietary advice given by medical professionals.

Emphasize eating smaller, more frequent meals to help with nutrient absorption and digestion. Meal plans should be minimal in fiber and easily digestible to reduce the possibility of irritants or obstructions. Cooking in batches could be useful if you're making bigger quantities of some dishes that you can save and reheat quickly throughout the week.

Try a variety of cooking techniques to determine which ones are most beneficial to your digestive system. Foods that are pureed or mashed can be easier to digest, and cooking methods like steaming, boiling, or baking may be kinder than frying.

CHAPTER THREE

DIETARY RECOMMENDATIONS FOR ILEOSTOMIES

HARMONIZING ELEMENTS

For those who have an ileostomy, eating a balanced diet is essential since it promotes overall health and well-being. To achieve nutrient balance, the intake of protein, carbs, fats, and fiber must be carefully considered. Protein is necessary for maintaining muscle mass and repairing tissue, and carbs offer a crucial source of energy. A variety of good fats, such as those in nuts, avocados, and olive oil, can assist meet a person's total nutritional needs.

When it comes to fiber, it's crucial to be aware of how much you eat because certain ileostomies may need to restrict their intake to avoid issues like intestinal obstructions. Prioritizing fiber sources that are simple to digest, including cooked veggies and peeled fruits, can ease digestive discomfort without sacrificing nutritional objectives. Finding the ideal mix that meets each person's demands and digestive tolerance may need routine monitoring and diet modifications.

TIPS FOR HYDRATION

Everyone needs to stay hydrated, but those who have an ileostomy need to be especially mindful of how much fluid they consume. Owing to the elevated danger of dehydration stemming from water loss via the stoma, it is advisable to ingest a sufficient quantity of fluids throughout the day. The most obvious and readily available alternative is water, but there are other hydrating options as well, such as clear soups, herbal teas, and electrolyte-rich beverages.

Hydration levels can be better managed by ingesting liquids gradually as opposed to in big quantities all at once. Urine color and frequency observations might be helpful markers of one's level of hydration. Additionally, modifying fluid intake becomes particularly crucial to make up for higher fluid losses during warmer weather or periods of greater physical activity. To assess each person's unique hydration requirements and make modifications in light of particular medical conditions and lifestyle choices, close collaboration with healthcare providers is important.

MINERALS AND VITAMINS

For those who have an ileostomy, maintaining an appropriate balance of vitamins and minerals is essential since the reconfiguration of the digestive system may cause changes in nutritional absorption. It is advised to regularly evaluate vitamin and mineral levels through blood tests to detect any potential deficits. To address particular nutrient demands, supplements could be required, and medical specialists can advise on the right amounts.

Iron, calcium, magnesium, vitamin B12, and calcium are some important vitamins and minerals to be aware of. Because the terminal ileum is the primary site of absorption for vitamin B12, deficits may need to be avoided by taking supplements. To prevent anemia, one must consume enough iron, and if dietary sources are inadequate, one may need to take supplements. The health of bones depends on calcium and magnesium, whose levels should be checked and supplementation should be considered if necessary.

A well-balanced diet that takes into account macronutrients, hydration, and vital vitamins and minerals can help people with ileostomies attain maximum nutritional health. To maintain long-term well-being and customize dietary suggestions to individual needs, collaboration with healthcare specialists is essential.

CHAPTER FOUR

MORNING TREATS

SMOOTHIES THAT INVIGORATE

Smoothies are becoming a popular option for breakfast lovers looking for a healthy and energizing way to start the day. These smoothies are made with a variety of fruits, veggies, and other healthful components to give you a quick energy boost. Energy-boosting smoothies, which include a range of nutrient-dense ingredients like berries, nuts, and leafy greens, are a revitalizing way to start your day. Incorporating components abundant in vitamins, minerals, and antioxidants not only improves taste but also supports general health. Smoothies are a popular choice for people who want to give their bodies a healthy dose of energy because of their adaptability to suit a variety of palates.

FILLING BREAKFAST BOWLS

Filling breakfast bowls have become a popular and adaptable breakfast choice for those with a variety of dietary needs. These bowls usually include a base consisting of grains, such as rice, quinoa, or oats, which give a substantial base. Protein options like eggs, Greek yogurt, or tofu give the dish solidity and make it a satisfying and healthful option. In addition, adding vibrant, nutrient-dense fruits and veggies, as well as toppings like nuts or seeds, not only improves the dish's appearance but also helps it to be well-balanced. Make breakfast a joyful and nutritious experience by experimenting with flavors and textures with hearty breakfast bowls, which serve as a canvas for creativity.

SIMPLE AND PACKED WITH NUTRIENTS

The need for quick and nutrient-dense breakfast options has increased in today's hectic environment as consumers look to maintain their health without sacrificing speed. These selections cover a wide range of alternatives, from quick-fix foods to simple meals. Smoothie packs that are already packaged, overnight oats, and energy bars are a few of the fast fixes that offer a nutrient boost in the least amount of time.

To provide a well-rounded lunch, these selections frequently combine a variety of nutritious grains, lean proteins, and important vitamins. Nutritional value is not compromised for convenience; instead, the emphasis is on providing the right nutrients for long-lasting energy in the morning. Modern lifestyles are catered to by the availability of such rapid and nutrient-dense solutions, which allow people to prioritize health without sacrificing valuable time in their hectic schedules.

CHAPTER FIVE

FAVORITES FOR LUNCH

SAVORY SALADS

Lunchtime favorites frequently offer a wide variety of tasty salads to suit different dietary requirements and palate preferences. These salads are a brilliant symphony of colors, textures, and tastes rather than merely a medley of greens. With their combination of crunchy, fresh veggies, fruits, nuts, and various meats, these salads make for a filling and healthy meal.

A well-balanced salad is mostly dependent on the quality of the dressing and the ingredients used. There are countless variations available, ranging from traditional Caesar salads made with romaine lettuce, croutons, and parmesan cheese to unique Mediterranean dishes made with olives, feta, and sun-dried tomatoes. Using components like grilled chicken, shrimp, or tofu, these salads frequently combine savory and sweet flavors to improve their overall palatability.

SANDWICHES AND WRAPS PACKED WITH PROTEIN

Sandwiches and wraps with lots of protein are favorite choices for people looking for a filling but quick lunch. Not only are these meals tasty, but they also supply the energy needed to go through the remainder of the day. These creations are stunning because they can be made to suit a wide range of nutritional requirements, including those of carnivores, vegetarians, and vegans.

These flavor-layered wraps and sandwiches are often packed with roast beef, turkey, grilled chicken, or vegetarian substitutes such as hummus or falafel. The ideal canvas is freshly made bread or wraps, to which creaminess and depth are added by toppings like avocado, cheese, and other spreads.

They are a great option for people who lead busy lifestyles or are just searching for a filling and delicious lunch option because they place a strong emphasis on protein, which guarantees a satisfying and fulfilling meal.

STEWS AND SOUPS

One nourishing and cozy type of lunchtime favorite is soups and stews, particularly in the winter months. These comforting and filling choices offer a source of nutrition that can be tailored to meet a variety of dietary needs and palate preferences in addition to being a visual and gustatory treat. You can find a wide range of options in this area, from thick chili to creamy tomato soup.

Soups and stews are popular because of their capacity to combine flavors through slow cooking, which lets components absorb and develop a unified flavor profile. These meals frequently achieve the ideal balance between heartiness and comfort, whether it's a rich and spicy gumbo with a smorgasbord of seafood or a chicken noodle soup packed with veggies. Soups and stews, served over rice or with crusty bread, provide a hearty and satisfying lunch that warms the body and the spirit.

CHAPTER SIX

DINNER IDEAS

HEALTHY ONE-POT DINNERS

The ease of use and harmony of flavors and textures that one-pot meals provide in a single cooking dish has made them extremely popular. The idea is to prepare well-balanced meals that include veggies, carbs, and proteins to make a satisfying and well-rounded meal. This method reduces the number of dishes that need to be cleaned while also enhancing the flavor depth when ingredients combine while cooking.

Making a well-balanced one-pot meal requires careful ingredient selection. A healthy balance of vital nutrients is ensured by including nutritious grains like brown rice or quinoa together with lean meats like chicken or tofu. Vegetables enhance the mixture with color, fiber, and several vitamins.

Herbs and seasonings are essential since they give the dish's flavor and depth. Hearty stews, casseroles, and skillet meals are a few examples of one-pot wonders that offer diversity and simplicity in preparation.

BAKED AND GRILLED SELECTIONS

Cooking methods like grilling and baking provide different ingredients with distinctive flavors and textures, which improves the dining experience. Fruits, vegetables, and meats all gain depth from the smoky, charred flavor that grilling gives.

Grilling caramelizes food, bringing out its inherent sweetness and resulting in a delicious flavor contrast. Grilled chicken, veggie skewers, or even fruit kebabs are all delicious options that bring a unique outdoor flavor to the dinner table.

However, baking is a more mild cooking technique that works well for foods that require a constant, uniform heat. Baked alternatives consist of roasted veggies, lasagna, and casseroles. Baking not only highlights an ingredient's inherent sweetness but also enables taste combinations to be combined creatively.

It's a flexible method that works well for savory as well as sweet foods, from filling dinners to decadent desserts.

PLANT-BASED AND VEGETARIAN RECIPES

Plant-based eating is becoming more and more popular, and this has led to a culinary revolution that has produced a wide range of delicious and nutrient-dense vegetarian and plant-based cuisine. Meals prepared for vegetarians emphasize plant-based protein sources such as beans, tofu, and tempeh combined with a wide variety of vegetables. These dishes highlight the variety of plant-based components and demonstrate that a diet devoid of meat can be just as flavorful and enjoyable as one that includes meat.

Plant-based recipes take things a step further by excluding all animal ingredients, such as dairy and eggs. Whole grains, nuts, seeds, and a plethora of fruits and vegetables are all welcome additions to this area.

These recipes, which highlight the advantages of a plant-based diet for both health and the environment, appeal to a wide range of palates and include inventive plant-based burgers, substantial lentil stews, and quinoa salads. The inventiveness with which flavors and textures are combined in plant-based and vegetarian cookery demonstrates a contemporary and environmentally conscious method of food preparation.

CHAPTER SEVEN

SIDES AND SNACKS

HEALTHY SNACK CONCEPTS

When it comes to nutritious snack options, finding a balance between taste and nutritional value is crucial. Nutrient-dense components guarantee that snacks not only satiate appetites but also have a good impact on general health. Snacks that include important vitamins and fiber include fresh fruits and vegetables like carrot sticks with hummus or apple slices with nut butter.

Another great option for maintaining energy levels throughout the day is snacks high in protein. A tasty and nutritious alternative is Greek yogurt topped with nuts or granola. A tiny portion of cottage cheese topped with cherry tomatoes or hard-boiled eggs are also excellent options since they provide a range of vital elements and protein.

When it comes to making snacks that are not only delicious but also high in complex carbs, whole grains are essential. Snack on cheese on wholegrain crackers or try herb-seasoned popcorn for a delightful crunch. These snacks are a great option for anyone looking for nutritional alternatives because they contribute to a sensation of fullness and provide prolonged energy.

DELICIOUS SIDE DISHES

With their complimentary flavors and textures, side dishes are a crucial component of any well-rounded dinner, elevating the whole eating experience. Delicious side dishes frequently have a well-balanced combination of components that go well with the main entrée. Broccoli infused with garlic or Brussels sprouts with a balsamic sauce are two examples of roasted veggies that give a platter a pop of color and taste.

Starchy side foods like quinoa pilaf or garlic mashed potatoes are substantial side dishes that provide the meal depth and satisfaction. A side dish that mixes the sweetness of corn with a burst of spiciness, like grilled corn on the cob with chili-lime butter, is a standout example.

Adding flavors from around the world to side dishes can improve the eating experience. For a delicious blend of flavors, try meals like Mexican street corn or couscous salad with herbs from the Mediterranean. These choices offer a gastronomic journey for the palate in addition to improving the dish.

CARRYING SNACKS FOR A MOVE

The necessity for portable snacks that we can eat on the go has grown in importance due to our fast-paced lifestyles. These snacks ought to be easy to transport and eat without sacrificing flavor or nutritional value. A traditional example of a portable snack with a pleasing crunch and a variety of flavors is a trail mix, which is a mixture of nuts, seeds, and dried fruits.

Whole-grain pita chips or pre-packaged hummus with vegetable sticks make a healthy and portable snack alternative. Furthermore, energy bars that are composed of healthy components like nuts, dried fruits, and oats provide a rapid energy boost without requiring refrigeration.

For a light and refreshing snack, prepackaged or bite-sized pieces of fresh fruit make great options. Apple slices, grapes, and berries are among the easily transportable fruits that are also hydrating and naturally sweet. Making sensible snack choices for on-the-go guarantees that those with hectic schedules may still eat a balanced and nutritious diet.

CHAPTER EIGHT

SWEETS FOR ALL OCCASIONS

SWEET TREATS THAT DON'T RISK YOUR HEALTH

Finding the perfect mix between decadence and health-conscious options has grown in significance when it comes to sweets. The idea of enjoying sweets without sacrificing health has inspired creative thinking in the food industry. Instead of giving in to the widespread belief that desserts are intrinsically harmful, home cooks and chefs are experimenting with different ingredients and cooking techniques to produce delicious desserts that don't make you feel guilty.

Making healthier sweets requires using natural sweeteners like agave nectar, maple syrup, or honey in place of refined sugar. This lowers the influence of glucose while also imparting a unique flavor profile. Incorporating whole grains and substitute flours, like coconut or almond flour, also adds nutrients without sacrificing the intended flavor and texture.

DESSERTS WITH FRUIT

Desserts made with fruit are a perfect example of how to combine the abundance of nature with creative cooking. By utilizing the inherent sweetness and vivid hues of fruits, these desserts provide a healthy and revitalizing substitute for customary sweets. The possibilities are as varied as the fruits themselves, ranging from delectable berry tarts to fascinating tropical fruit salads.

Fruit-based sweets have a notable benefit in that they are quite versatile. Fruits can be added to food in a variety of ways, such as fresh slices, purees, or compotes, to enhance the dish's texture and appearance. In addition to tasting delicious, these treats are packed with nutritional benefits, including vital vitamins, antioxidants, and dietary fiber.

Fruit-based sweets are a popular choice for both informal get-togethers and formal festivities due to their ease of preparation and capacity to highlight seasonal food.

LUXURIOUS OCCASIONAL TREATS

Though the search for healthier dessert options is admirable, indulging in rich desserts once in a while has a distinct place in the world of gastronomic delights. Occasional indulgences in decadence are often associated with festivities, commemorating achievements, and fostering lifelong memories. Rich, opulent ingredients like butter, milk, and chocolate are frequently used in these sweets, taking the sensory experience to a whole new level of decadence.

These delicacies, which range from delicately layered chocolate cakes to silky custards and smooth tiramisu, are expertly made with care and accuracy. The secret to getting the right texture and depth of taste is using premium ingredients. These decadent confections act as a centerpiece, enticing the senses and evoking an air of richness, rather than just being a sweet way to end a meal.

The selection of desserts for all occasions is changing to meet the needs of a wide range of dietary restrictions and tastes. The current dessert menu offers a variety of options to suit different tastes and times, whether one is looking to indulge occasionally in extravagance, explore the colorful world of fruit-based delights, or prefer sweets without sacrificing health.

CHAPTER NINE

ORGANIZING EVENTS THAT ARE ILEOSTOMY-FRIENDLY

It takes careful planning to host events in a way that makes it welcoming and comfortable for people with ileostomies. An ileostomy is a surgical technique that allows waste to be eliminated by redirecting the small intestine through a stoma or opening in the belly. Organizing events that are ileostomy-friendly requires taking into account the special requirements and worries of those who have this condition.

One important thing to think about is accessibility to restrooms. Making sure there is a discreet and conveniently located bathroom can make a big difference in how comfortable visitors with ileostomies feel. Giving people access to basic materials like inconspicuous disposal bins and bags can help them handle their demands confidently and covertly.

It's important to consider any dietary limitations related to ileostomy treatment when organizing the gathering's meal. Choosing foods that are low in fiber and readily digested can be advantageous because they are generally easier on the digestive tract. Furthermore, offering a range of options—such as gluten-free and vegetarian options—guarantees that everyone may enjoy the meal without worrying about causing digestive problems.

To ensure that people with ileostomies may sit comfortably and without feeling self-conscious, seating arrangements should also be taken into account. Having pillows or cozy chairs can improve the whole experience for visitors, letting them unwind and take in the company without having to worry about being uncomfortable.

Additionally, communication is essential. To make sure you are ready to accommodate your ileostomy guests, gently enquire about any special requirements or preferences they may have. Fostering a culture of understanding and openness encourages diversity and makes the event fun for all attendees.

RECIPES FOR HOLIDAYS & CELEBRATIONS

Holidays and celebrations frequently revolve around delectable foods that unite people. It takes a combination of tradition, imagination, and careful attention to detail to create recipes that will be remembered for these unique events. There are many dishes available that may make any party more spectacular, from festive appetizers to decadent sweets.

To begin with, think about providing distinct and tasty appetizers that establish the mood for the event. A tasty way to start a meal, appetizers can include anything from little bruschettas to decadent cheese platters or stuffed mushrooms with flavorful stuffing.

Traditional Christmas roasts like turkey, ham, or roast beef are great options for main dishes. On the other hand, experimenting with different flavors and cooking methods can give the dish a contemporary edge. You can add something new and interesting to the table by marinating meats in unusual sauces, roasting them with aromatic herbs, or trying out different international cuisines.

Sides are essential to completing the festive meal. Traditional fare like stuffing, cranberry sauce, and mashed potatoes are mainstays, but creative sides like sweet potato casserole with a pecan crust or roasted Brussels sprouts with balsamic glaze may bring in new tastes and textures.

Desserts are the big conclusion of any party, and there are plenty of options for those who enjoy sweets. Dessert spreads can range from classic pies like pumpkin and pecan to rich cakes and cookies, showcasing a wide variety of flavors. To give your baked goods a Christmas feel, try adding seasonal ingredients like ginger, nutmeg, and cinnamon.

CHAPTER TEN

ADVICE FOR DINING OUT AND VACATIONING

DINING OUT WITH SELF-ASSUREDNESS

Making healthy food choices and interpreting menus when dining out might be difficult at times, but with a few thoughtful techniques, you can eat with confidence. If at all feasible, start your research on the restaurant beforehand. These days, a lot of places offer their menus online so you may look over your options and decide what to want before you go. Look for nutritional data, dietary labels, or reviews that may provide information about the healthier options on the menu.

Ask your server any queries you may have about the preparation techniques or any ingredient substitutions once you're at the restaurant. Dietary restrictions are typically accommodated, and staff members are frequently able to suggest healthier options. Instead of frying, choose baked, steamed, or grilled foods; also, pay attention to portion amounts. If the servings are huge, think about splitting a meal or requesting a half piece.

When dining out, another method to choose healthier options is to go for herbal teas or water instead of sugary drinks. Alcohol consumption should also be considered carefully since it can include empty calories. To stay hydrated, consider lighter drinks or switch to water if you must have one.

Finally, enjoy your food by eating mindfully of your body's signals and taking your time. Rather than overindulging, pay attention to your hunger and fullness cues and quit eating when you're satisfied. When you approach eating out with mindfulness and awareness, it can be a fun experience that still supports your health objectives.

TRAVEL-FRIENDLY RECIPES & TIPS

Maintaining a nutritious diet when traveling might present special obstacles, but you can prioritize nutrition while on the go with a little preparation and wise decision-making. Carry nutrient-dense foods with you on your travels, such as granola bars, almonds, and seeds. These foods can help stave off hunger between meals and are convenient and non-perishable.

Choose healthier options like salads, grilled proteins, and fresh fruit when dining at airports or rest areas. Nowadays, a lot of airports provide a range of food options, including healthier substitutes for classic fast food. If you can, try packing some salads or sandwiches of your own to cut down on the amount of time you spend eating at the airport or on the road.

When traveling, it's important to stay hydrated, so bring a reusable water bottle and fill it up frequently. Hydration should always come first because dehydration can cause weariness and hunger. Reducing alcohol and caffeine intake is also recommended because they can exacerbate dehydration.

Make use of any facilities offered by the hotel, such as the microwave and mini-fridge. This lessens your reliance on less wholesome options by enabling you to make and store some basic, healthful meals or snacks in your room.

Enjoy the food of the place you are visiting while paying attention to portion quantities. Choose dishes that are grilled or steamed, and make sure your meals contain a range of veggies. One satisfying method to enhance the nutritional worth of your trip is to explore local markets for fresh food.

Eating out and traveling may be pleasant without sacrificing your dedication to a healthy lifestyle if you prepare ahead and make thoughtful decisions.